YOUR KNOWLEDGE HAS VALUE

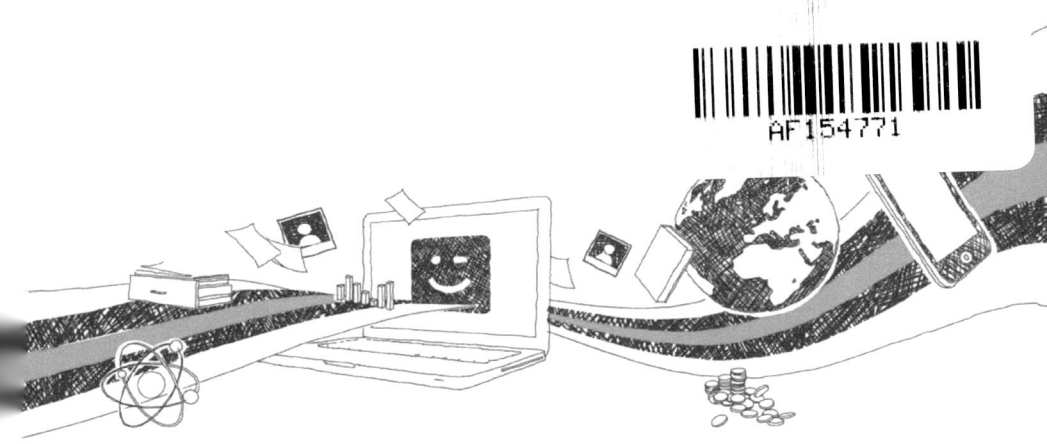
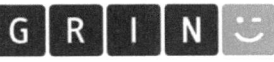

Charles Ross

Metabolic syndrome

GRIN Verlag

Bibliografische Information der Deutschen Nationalbibliothek:

Die Deutsche Bibliothek verzeichnet diese Publikation in der Deutschen National-
bibliografie; detaillierte bibliografische Daten sind im Internet über http://dnb.d-
nb.de/ abrufbar.

Imprint:

Copyright © 2010 GRIN Verlag GmbH
Druck und Bindung: Books on Demand GmbH, Norderstedt Germany
ISBN: 978-3-656-61073-1

This book at GRIN:

http://www.grin.com/en/e-book/269787/metabolic-syndrome

GRIN - Your knowledge has value

Der GRIN Verlag publiziert seit 1998 wissenschaftliche Arbeiten von Studenten, Hochschullehrern und anderen Akademikern als eBook und gedrucktes Buch. Die Verlagswebsite www.grin.com ist die ideale Plattform zur Veröffentlichung von Hausarbeiten, Abschlussarbeiten, wissenschaftlichen Aufsätzen, Dissertationen und Fachbüchern.

Visit us on the internet:

http://www.grin.com/

http://www.facebook.com/grincom

http://www.twitter.com/grin_com

Metabolic Syndrome: Teaching Nurses To Identify At Risk Patients

Acknowledgements

I am thankful to the Almighty God for directing me through an exciting and satisfying journey. I am also grateful of Dr. Jane Hibbert for guidance and offering support. Last but not the least, I am very proud to be part of a family that regards and motivates me to be the best I can be.

ABSTRACT

Formerly known as Problem X or Blood insulin Proof Problem, Metabolic syndrome is a number of metabolic risks, which can lead to one having high chance of creating heart problems, heart stroke, side-line general illness, and type-2 diabetic issues (Hurst pg. 86,2010. Detecting metabolic syndrome is a process that has been the middle of questionable conversation by Healthcare groups such as the World Health Organization (WHO), and other physicians. Conversations such as analytic requirements and therapy continue to cause warmed controversy due to the complexness of the actual cause of the differential analysis, but insulin level of resistance and being overweight are considered key elements (Calhoun, pg.90, 2011). In 1999, the World Health Organization described metabolic syndrome as, insulin level of resistance, sugar intolerance or incapacity, and being overweight. Later, in 2006, the Western Team for the Research of Blood insulin Resistance described metabolic syndrome by using going on a fast blood sugar stages to determine insulin level of resistance and provided factors for high blood pressure, triglyceride stages, HDL-C stages, and central being overweight by calculating hips area. In more recent reports, cultural background and genes play an essential part for the analysis of metabolic syndrome (Weiss, pg. 87, 2012). Another study conducted by the National Cholesterol Education Program Third Adult Treatment Board modified in 2005, set five specific requirements and cutoffs than previously described (Byrne, pg97, 2011). Healthcare experts nationwide use this standard as a basis to identify a person with metabolic syndrome if three of the five requirements are met

CHAPTER 1

2

Metabolic Problem is a group of cardio-metabolic threats, such as obesity, hyperglycemia, dyslipidemia and great blood vessels stress, and has been connected with raised chance of creating Center Illness and Kind 2 Diabetic issues. It is approximated that approximately 39% of the US mature inhabitants meets the requirements for Metabolic Problem. The aim of this project was to assess the role of positive diagnosis of Metabolic Problem on Medical care Usage – specifically on the annual variety of hospitalizations and physician's trips to the doctor. Data on 16,632 topics was produced from the Third Nationwide Wellness and Nutrition Evaluation Survey dataset and used for research (Abdul-Rahim, pg. 87, 2011). It was determined from Multivariate Multiple Regression model that the variety of Hospitalizations and Doctors Workplace trips is considerably greater in topics with Metabolic Problem bookkeeping for variations in age, race and gender. It was also seen that the factors selected for research included a very portion of the difference in variety of hospitalizations and physician's trips to the doctor. It was hence determined that further work was required to assess the influence of Metabolic Problem on healthcare utilization while bookkeeping for these unknown aspects (Das,pg100,2010).

1. Introduction

Metabolic Problem is a group of cardio-metabolic threats that has shown to considerably improve the chance of creating Center Illness and Kind 2 Diabetic issues Mellitus. Threat aspects consist of stomach obesity, hyperglycemia (elevated blood vessels glucose), and dyslipidemias (abnormal blood vessels fat levels) and great blood vessels stress elevated blood vessels pressure. It is approximated that 2500 People in America die from CVD each day with costs related to CVD approximating to $403 billion dollars yearly (Batone,pg97,2008).

Fat

What is metabolic syndrome? According to the U.S Department of health and Human Services, Metabolic Problem is the name "for a group of threats aspects connected to

3

overweight and obesity that improve your chance for cardiovascular disease and other health problems". Human extra fat is much more than "just a layer of insulating material or something we wish we had less of". As a point actually, the quantity of fat your human body contains can actually impact wellbeing. Therefore, Scientists have been offering us with ideas that can provide us signs to important illnesses and conditions (Vinik, pg. 87, 2012).

The quantity of fat and the way it is distributed inside our bodies seem to be significant   signs of the metabolic problems. When the following signs are available in a mixture of three or more, the individual has the metabolic syndrome. The signs listed here are: raised triglycerides, blood insulin level of resistance, great blood vessels stress, central stomach obesity and low great density lip necessary protein. An amazing reality in this passage is that twenty four percent of the mature inhabitants has metabolic syndrome.

Some of the adipocytes identified here are: Leptin, Resistin, Visfatin, and Adniponectin. There are many others but some of them remain unknown at this present. The next few sections give a useful description of each of the adipocytes. For example, Visfatin is known to be just like blood insulin, Lepton allows reduce appetite and so forth.

Metabolic syndrome is a mixture of medical conditions that improve the chance of creating cardiovascular disease and diabetes. It impacts one in five individuals, and occurrence increases with age. Some studies calculate the occurrence in the USA to be up to 25% of the inhabitants.

Metabolic syndrome is also known as metabolic syndrome X, syndrome X, blood insulin level of resistance syndrome, Reaven's syndrome, and CHAOS (Australia)[3]. A identical condition in overweight horse is referred to as horse metabolic

History

The phrase "metabolic syndrome" goes back to at least the delayed Nineteen fifties, but came into typical usage in 4 decades ago to explain various organizations of threats with diabetes that had been mentioned as early as the Twenties.

4

The Marseilles doctor Dr. Jean Unexplained, in 1947, observed that breasts obesity appeared to predispose to diabetes, heart disease, gouty arthritis, and calculi.

Avogaro, Crepaldi and co-workers described six somewhat overweight patients with diabetes, hypercholesterolemia, and marked hypertriglyceridemia all of which improved when the patients were put on a hypocaloric, low carbs eating plan.

In 1977, Haller used the phrase "metabolic syndrome" for organizations of obesity, diabetes mellitus, hyperlipoproteinemia, hyperuricemia and Hepatic steatosis when explaining the preservative effects of threats on heart disease (Milionis, pg87, 2012).

The same year, Musician used the phrase for organizations of obesity, gouty arthritis, diabetes mellitus, and great blood vessels stress with hyperlipoprotenemia.

In 1977 and 1978, Gerald B. Phillips developed the concept that threats for myocardial infarction recognize to form a "constellation of abnormalities" (i.e., sugar intolerance, hyperinsulinemia, hyperlipidemia [hypercholesterolemia and hypertriglyceridemia] and hypertension) that is associated not only with cardiovascular disease, but also with aging, obesity and other clinical declares.

These days, it is not amazing that junk meals projects and restaurants are offering almost all our population's eating plan. Along with the busy plans and unhealthy dining, we as individuals are not as physically dedicated to maintaining a work out commitment or a weight loss program plan routine. Therefore, almost all People in America are suffering from an illness called Metabolic Problem.

Metabolic Problem is typical in individuals that are older in age, postmenopausal, tobacco users, consume great carbs food, and live a inactive lifestyle with little to no work out (Brown, 2011, pg. 442). The circumstances found in the course publication were very typical to what our entire inhabitants' experiences with and in most occasions develop into different and greater risk illnesses.

The circumstances of Metabolic Problem consist of heart illnesses to consist of

5

hyperinsulenemia, which places an individual at a risky for heart, heart stroke, and type- 2 diabetes (Brown, 2011, pg. 442). In addition to heart issues, Metabolic Problem impacts an individual's great blood vessels stress, blood sugar stages, good and bad cholesterols, such as raised triglycerides. Most individuals also have stomach obesity (Brown, 2011, pg. 442). In order for researching prospective substitute drugs and natural herbs, the Nationwide Center for Supporting and Alternative Medicine allows promote and fund grants to Colleges. To assess the potency of botanicals in regards to circumstances such as great blood vessels stress, cardiovascular disease, intellectual decrease, blood insulin level of resistance, and excess fats in the blood vessels, NCCAM financed researchers at the University of The state of Creole at Manchester to conduct a literary works review and examine and study from their own lab.

Metabolic issue is a cluster of conditions — increased high blood pressure, a higher glucose level, undesirable personal additional fat around the waist and abnormal blood veins cholesterol levels — that occur together, increasing your possibility of middle sickness, middle heart stroke and being suffering from diabetes.

Having just one of these conditions doesn't mean you have metabolic issue. However, any of these conditions enhance your possibility of serious sickness. If more than one of these conditions occur in combination, your risk is even higher (Blaha pg98, 2012).

If you have metabolic issue or any of the components of metabolic issue, aggressive way of lifestyle changes can delay or even prevent the development of serious health problems Metabolic issue is a collection of disorders that occur together and enhance your possibility of developing type two being suffering from diabetes or heart attack (stroke or middle disease). The causes of metabolic issue are complex and not well understood, but there is thought to be a genetic link. Being overweight or overweight and physically inactive adds to your risk. Metabolic issue is sometimes called issue X or insulin-resistance issue.

As we get older, we tend to become less active and may gain additional human bodyweight.

This human bodyweight is generally stored around the abdomen. This can lead to the whole human body becoming up against the hormone blood veins blood insulin. This means that blood veins blood insulin in one's personal is less effective, especially in the muscles and liver human body organ.

More than 25 per cent of Australian adults have metabolic issue. This is higher in people with being suffering from diabetes.

A group of conditions that occur together

Metabolic issue is not a sickness in itself, but a collection of risks for that often occur together. A personal is classed as having metabolic issue when they have any three or more of:

Primary (abdominal) obesity – undesirable fat in and around the abdomen (abdomen)

Raised high blood pressure (hypertension)

Great veins triglycerides

Low stages of great stability lipoproteins (HDL) – the 'good' cholesterol

Affected going on a quick glucose (IFG) or being suffering from diabetes. IFG happens when veins glucose stages levels are uncommonly great, but not sufficient to be diagnosed as type two being suffering from diabetes.

Insulin resistance

Insulin level of level of resistance means that your whole human body does not use the hormone blood veins blood insulin as effectively as it should, especially in the muscles and liver human body organ.

Normally, your digestive tract breaks down carbohydrates into glucose, which then passes from your intestine into your veins. As your veins glucose stages level rises, your pancreatic secretes blood veins blood insulin into your veins. Insulin allows glucose to move into your muscle cells from your veins. Once inside a cell, the glucose is 'burned' – along with oxygen – to produce energy.

When a personal has blood veins blood insulin level of level of resistance, the pancreatic needs to release more blood veins blood insulin than usual to maintain regular veins glucose stages levels. It is thought that more than a quarter of the population has some degree of level of potential to deal with blood veins blood insulin.

The link to diabetes

Insulin level of level of resistance enhances your possibility of developing type two being suffering from diabetes and is found in most people with this type of being suffering from diabetes. If the pancreatic can't produce additional blood veins blood insulin to overcome your human body level of level of resistance, your veins glucose stages levels will rise and you will develop affected going on a quick glucose, affected glucose tolerance (IGT) or being suffering from diabetes. Those who type two being suffering from diabetes frequently also have other features of metabolic issue and a significantly increased possibility of middle (heart and veins vessel) sickness.

Central obesity

Central obesity is when the primary deposits of personal additional fat are around the abdomen and the breasts. The higher your waist circumference, the higher your risk. A person's risk for main obesity varies depending on their gender and social background. As a general rule, if your waist measures 94 cm or more (men) or 80 cm or more (women), you probably need to lose some human bodyweight. Men from Middle Eastern, South Oriental, Chinese, Asian-Indian, South and Primary American social backgrounds are considered at risk if their waist measures 90 cm or more.

High blood pressure (hypertension)

In the absence of other risks, high blood pressure happens when a personal has a high blood pressure higher than 140/90mmHg. This may be due to genetics, way of lifestyle or other diseases such as kidney or heart attack. Hypertension also enhances your possibility of developing heart attack, middle heart stroke and kidney sickness.

The ideal high blood pressure range is less than 130/80 mmHg (or lower, if other diseases are present), but everyone is different. Check with your doctor to find the right target for you and make sure your high blood pressure is checked regularly.

Lifestyle changes such as regular training, not cigarette smoking cigarettes, reducing the amount of sodium (salt) in your diet, reducing stress, limiting alcohol and achieving health weight may help, but sometimes drugs is required.

Cholesterol and triglycerides

Cholesterol is a harmful substance that we make in our liver human body organ. LDL (low stability lipoproteins) cholesterol levels can block bloodstream by building up on the walls of veins. HDL (high stability lipoproteins) cholesterol levels help protect against this build-up of harmful blockages.

Triglycerides may come from foods we eat, but they are also produced by the liver human body organ. Drinking undesirable alcohol can contribute to a rise in triglycerides. If you are blood veins blood insulin resistant, you are likely to have higher-than-normal triglyceride stages. Great veins triglycerides tend to be associated with low stages of HDL cholesterol levels – the 'good' or protective cholesterol levels.

Raised triglycerides and reduced HDL cholesterol levels enhance your risk for heart (narrowing of the arteries), which is a contributing factor in middle sickness. Overweight or obesity is also a risk factor in itself for conditions such as great triglyceride stages, great high blood pressure and heart.

Impaired glucose tolerance (pre-diabetes)

Impaired going on a quick glucose and affected glucose tolerance are sometimes referred to as 'pre-diabetes'. They happen when your veins glucose stages level is uncommonly great, but not sufficient to be called being suffering from diabetes. One third of people who have affected glucose tolerance or affected going on a quick glucose will develop being suffering from diabetes unless way of lifestyle changes are made.

Does one condition induce the others?

All of these conditions are interlinked in complicated ways and it is difficult to work out the chain of events. Which condition – if any – is the primary trigger? Some researchers consider that obesity could be the starting point for the metabolic issue.

Reducing your human bodyweight and participating in regular training may enhance your triglyceride and blood veins cholesterol levels, lower your high blood pressure and enhance your human body response to blood veins blood insulin. This may help prevent you from developing type two being suffering from diabetes and heart attack.

Ways to reduce your risk

More than half of all Australians have at least one of the metabolic issue conditions. Suggestions for reducing your risk include:

Incorporate as many positive way of lifestyle changes as you can – eating weight loss programs, training and reducing human bodyweight will dramatically reduce your possibility of diseases associated with metabolic issue, such as being suffering from diabetes and middle sickness.

Make dietary changes – eat plenty of natural wholegrain foods, vegetables and fruit. To help with losing human bodyweight, reduce the amount of food you eat and limit foods rich in fat or glucose. Reduce fats, which are present in meat, full-cream dairy and many harmful foods. Stop alcohol consumption or reduce your intake to less than two standard drinks a day.

Enhance your training level – actual exercise can take many different forms according to what suits you best. Try and do at least 30 minutes of exercise on at least five days of each week. Also try to avoid spending prolonged periods of time sitting down, by standing up or going for a one-to-two minute walk.

Manage your human bodyweight – increasing training and improving dietary habits will help you lose undesirable personal additional fat, and reduce your human bodyweight.

Stop cigarette smoking cigarettes – cigarette smoking cigarettes enhances your possibility of heart attack, middle heart stroke, and cancer and lung sickness. Quitting will have many benefits, especially if you have metabolic issue (Iacobellis,pg97,2009).

Medication may be required – way of lifestyle changes is very important in the management of the metabolic issue, but sometimes drugs may be necessary to manage the different conditions. Some people will need to take antihypertensive tablets to control great high blood pressure or lipid-lowering medications (or both) to keep cholesterol levels within the recommended limits. The most essential thing is to reduce your possibility of heart attack, being suffering from diabetes and middle heart stroke (Isaacs, pg95, 2010).

Check with your doctor to decide what the best management strategy is for you.

CHAPTER 3: REVIEW OF LITERATURE

A preliminary search was conducted using MEDLINE, OVID, , CINAHL, and Cochrane data source. Information collection was produced by using search phrases such as: wellness professional residence, new graduate student wellness professional storage, wellness professional internship, new wellness professional attrition, and new wellness professional proficiency.

Formerly known as Issue X or Blood insulin Proof Issue, Metabolic syndrome is a number of metabolic threats, which can lead to one having high chance of creating heart problems, heart stroke, side-line general illness, and type-2 diabetic issues. Detecting metabolic syndrome is a process that has been the middle of questionable conversation by Healthcare groups such as the Center for Disease Control (CDC), the Globe Health Company (WHO), and other physicians. Conversations such as analytic requirements and therapy continue to cause warmed controversy due to the complexness of the actual cause of the differential analysis, but insulin level of resistance and being overweight are considered key elements. In 1999, the Globe Health Company described metabolic syndrome as, insulin level of resistance, sugar intolerance or incapacity, and being overweight. Later, in 2006, the Western Team for the Research of Blood insulin Resistance (EGIR) described metabolic syndrome by using going

11

on a fast blood sugar stages to determine insulin level of resistance and provided factors for high blood pressure, triglyceride stages, HDL-C stages, and central being overweight by calculating hips area. In more recent reports, cultural background and genes perform an essential part for the analysis of metabolic syndrome. Another study conducted by the National Cholesterol levels Education Program Third Adult Treatment Board modified in 2005, set five specific requirements and cutoffs than previously described. Healthcare experts nationwide use this standard as a basis to identify a person with metabolic syndrome if three of the five requirements are met.

CHAPTER 4: METHODOLOGY

This illustrative design study is designed at increasing attention of nurses' information concerning metabolic syndrome and the part they perform on strengthening at threat sufferers by teaching them on metabolic syndrome. This chapter will deal with the summary of the issue and the techniques to carry out the venture.

Approximately 55 million people in the United States, or 1 out of 3 People in America over the age of 20, with the majority being Africa and Spanish American females more than men, are affected by metabolic syndrome and may not be aware of their medical threats until an actual problem occur. The disproportion of females to men is said to be connected to the amount of adipose tissue females are susceptible to, the difference in cholesterol information between men and ladies, raised triglycerides are more highly associated with heart in females than in men, and aspects unique to females such as polycystic-ovary syndrome, hormone birth control pill use, and gestational diabetic issues, are threats. It was also once thought that most sufferers with metabolic syndrome also have kind two diabetic issues, but current results show that metabolic syndrome preserves its value for heart results even in the lack of kind two diabetic issues.

IRB acceptance will be posted. IRB recommendations were followed to secure members and data. The next stage is why an academic in-service would help deal with the issue. The academic in-service will evaluate the preliminary understanding of nursing staff and help recognize at threat sufferers for academic resources. To recognize at threat individual's nursing staff will be knowledgeable about the issue, occurrence, threats and course of action associated with metabolic syndrome (Bagchi, pg86, 2012).

Prior to the in-service a 10 item evaluation device will be applied to volunteers. This evaluation device was designed based on the review of literary works defined in this offer. Approximately 55 thousand people in the U. s. Declares, or 1 out of 3 People in America over the age of 20, with the majority being Africa and Spanish U. s. states females more than men, are suffering from metabolic problem and may not be aware of their medical threats until an actual problem occur. The disproportion of females to men is said to be connected to the amount of adipose cells females are susceptible to, the difference in cholesterol levels information between men and ladies, raised triglycerides are more highly associated with heart in females than in men, and aspects unique to females such as polycystic-ovary problem, hormone birth control pill use, and gestational diabetic issues, are threats. It was also once thought that most sufferers with metabolic problem also have kind two diabetic issues, but present results show that metabolic problem preserves its value for heart results even in the lack of kind two diabetic issues.

Purpose

The objective of this illustrative design study is to present literary works less than five years old that describes the significant effect metabolic problem is having on sufferers and to inform the inhabitants about the occurrence of and how to decrease threats for metabolic problem.

Significance Statement

Review of recent literary works reviews that metabolic problem enhances the chance of heart results and almost enhances as the cause of death rate. There is restricted information and a gap in cultural analysis available on the occurrence of metabolic problem, but education and

13

learning is a key factor in decreasing the chance of being impacted.   Avoidance and decrease of metabolic problem is essential to decrease cardiac arrest and to boost life in the mature inhabitants.

Research Question

The aim of this document is to explain the present understanding of medical nursing staff regarding metabolic problem occurrence, threats and problems.

A diagnosis of metabolic problem is made if a person has any three of the following threat factors:

Waist circumference: at least 35 inches wide for females and at least 40 inches wide for men.

Fasting blood vessels blood glucose stages at least 100 mg/dL

Serum triglycerides at least 150 mg/dL

Blood pressure at least 135/85mmHg

HDL ("good") cholestrerol stages decreased than 40 mg/dL for men or 50 mg/dL for women

Metabolic Syndrome seems to impact between 25 and 30 % of the U.S. inhabitants according to various national health surveys. In fact, the amount of people with metabolic problem seems to improve as we get older, affecting four in 10 Americans as they reach their 60s and 70s.

What are the symptoms?

Usually, there are no immediate physical signs. People with metabolic problem do have a tendency to be overweight, especially around the abdomen - having an "apple shape." Moreover, since this condition is associated with blood vessels insulin level of resistance, those with metabolic problem may display some of the medical functions associated with a rise in the production of blood vessels insulin. For instance, females may experience cysts on their ovaries (metabolic problem is associated with polycystic ovarian syndrome) and irregular periods. People can have an increased occurrence of epidermis tags, benign raised growths of epidermis that usually appear improves on the spinal.Consistently great stages of blood vessels insulin are associated with many harmful changes in the whole body prior to its manifesting as illness including chronic swelling and harm to arterial walls, decreased excretion of salt by the kidneys, and thickening of the blood vessels. People with metabolic problem also display levels in hypertension and changes in their blood vessels lipids, primarily with triglycerides (elevated) and good cholesterol levels or great density lipoprotein (HDL) (reduced). Problems associated with metabolic problem develop over time and usually worsen if neglected.

What are the causes?

The exact cause of metabolic problem is unknown. It is frequently influenced by living, but also seems to be genetically driven. As stated, many functions of metabolic problem are associated with "insulin level of resistance," which causes tissues to reduce their sensitivity to blood vessels insulin; the hormonal needed to allow blood vessels blood glucose stages to enter tissues for use as fuel. As blood glucose stages in the blood vessels improve, the pancreas tries to overcompensate and produce even more blood vessels insulin, which ultimately outcomes in the characteristic signs of metabolic problem. When stages of blood vessels insulin spike, a pressure response occurs that outcomes in levels in cortisol, your long-acting pressure hormonal. This in turn creates an inflammation related reaction that if remaining unchecked begins to harm healthier tissue (Redmon,pg87,2012).

Interestingly enough, some data suggests that consumption of sodas (diet or regular) and other items containing high-fructose corn syrup (HFCS) like treatments and ketchup, jams, jellies, ice cream and many more foods may be connected to obesity, blood vessels insulin level of resistance, and metabolic problem in people of all ages. Interrupted rest patterns (such as rest apnea) may also be a factor in increasing the occurrence of blood vessels insulin level of resistance and metabolic problem in the adult inhabitants.

What is the traditional treatment?

The main goal of medical management is to decrease cardiovascular risks and prevent type two diabetic issues. The major risks for cardiac illness consist of cigarette smoking cigarettes, blood vessels lipid abnormalities, hypertension and glucose, all of which should be decreased to recommended stages. Aggressive way of life changes, and in some cases drugs, can improve most if not all components of metabolic problem.

Moderate losing bodyweight, in the variety of 5 to ten % of bodyweight, can help restore your ability to recognize blood vessels insulin and decrease the chance of developing diabetic issues. It will also decrease hypertension and cholesterol levels. Fitness such as a brisk 30-minute everyday walk can be impressive in enhancing stages of blood vessels insulin, facilitating losing bodyweight, and enhancing related signs. Most experts suggest 30-60 minutes every day of average intensity work out on at least five days per 7 days either divided throughout the day or all at once; the same benefit is achieved either way.

Most traditional experts suggest that sufferers adhere to a diet plan like the American Nutritional Association diet plan, the Nutritional Approaches to Stop Hypertension diet plan or the Mediterranean Diet. All of these emphasize fruits, vegetables, and whole grain, while limiting bad body fat and promoting leaner important like low-fat dairy and liver organ like chicken and seafood.

A main intervention for metabolic problem is to initiate cigarettes programs. Smoking cigarettes improves blood vessels insulin level of resistance and worsens the health consequences of metabolic problem.

Doctors may also prescribe medications to decreased hypertension, control cholesterol levels or help you shed bodyweight. Insulin sensitizers like Glucophage (Metformin) may be prescribed to help your whole body use blood vessels insulin more effectively. It lowers blood vessels blood glucose stages, which also seems to help decreased cholesterol levels levels and triglycerides as well as decreasing appetite. The adverse reactions of Metformin (often temporary) consist of nausea, stomach pain, bloating and diarrhea. A more serious complication, lactic acidosis, can impact those with kidney or liver illness, severe center

16

failure or a history of excessive drinking and is possibly, though rarely, fatal. Aspirin therapy is often given to help decrease chance of cardiac problems.

What therapies does Dr. Weil suggest for metabolic syndrome?

Dietary changes: The traditional medical recommendation of a low-fat, high-carbohydrate diet plan to decreased triglycerides and bring down cholesterol levels is dead incorrect in his opinion. Consuming a weight loss program plan great in the incorrect kinds of carbs and fat may actually increase triglycerides and cholesterol levels. Instead, Dr. Weil suggests following an anti-inflammatory diet plan. This is a not a weight loss program plan in the popular sense - it is not intended as a weight-loss program (although people can and do shed bodyweight on it), nor is it an diet plan to stay on for a limited time period. Rather, it is way of selecting and preparing foods based on scientific knowledge of how they can help your whole body remain optimally healthier. Along with influencing swelling, the diet plan will provide steady energy and ample vitamins, minerals, fat and soluble fiber. The following suggestions incorporate the principles of this way of eating:

Eat small, frequent foods to keep blood vessels blood glucose stages in a proper and balanced variety. Consuming huge foods can flood the bloodstream with glucose and blood vessels insulin. Experiment until you find that you feel your best.

Keep refined starches and sugars to a lowest, instead choosing those with a low list. (Sweet potatoes, winter crush and legumes are examples of better carbohydrates.) You should also be aware of glycemic load in assessing dietary choices (Athyros,pg98,2011).

Keep body fat and trans-fats to a lowest, but consume average quantities of monounsaturated sebum, such as olive oil and some nut sebum.

Eat seafood several times per 7 days, emphasizing wild, cold-water seafood great in omega-3 human extra fat, such as salmon and sardines. Or take omega-3 items.

Eat generous quantities of non-starchy vegetables, like cucumbers, peppers, green greens, zucchini, eggplant, crush, asparagus, broccoli, cabbage, Brussels sprouts, legumes, radishes

17

and green spinach.

Eat foods great in mineral magnesium, which research has connected to lowering the occurrence of metabolic problem. One gets mineral magnesium by consuming plenty of whole grain, vegetables (spinach is a great source) as well as almonds, cashews and other nuts, avocados, legumes, soybeans, and halibut.

Cut returning on liquor, avoiding beer especially. (Even little liquor can increase triglyceride stages.)

For more information on the anti-inflammatory diet plan, check out Dr. Weil's Anti-Inflammatory Food Pyramid.

Exercise: Getting exercising is vital but too a lot of people quit, become injured, or simply find the process less enjoyable than they should. Follow Dr. Weil's advice for making cardio exercise work out an ongoing, secure and rewarding part of your life.

Mind/Body: It is important to attend to pressure in positive methods. Rather than using liquor, tobacco, or television, try breathing exercises. They are simple, free, and right under your nose. Dr. Weil has compiled ten methods peace and promotes relaxation, calm and peace within you. Some techniques take practice, and most require some commitment on your part to achieve outcomes. However, the outcomes are well worth the effort.

Supplements:

An antioxidant complement and multivitamin-mineral complement.

You can take additional mineral magnesium if you do not think you're getting enough in the diet plan. Dr. Weil suggests mineral magnesium citrate, chelate, or glycine. Avoid mineral magnesium oxide, which can be irritating, and take half the amount of mineral magnesium as the calcium mineral you take in additional type. If you do not take any additional calcium mineral, watch out for getting considerable quantities of mineral magnesium, which can cause diarrhea.

If you are avoiding oily seafood at least twice per 7 days, take additional seafood oil, in

18

capsule or liquid type, 1-2 grams a day. Look for molecularly distilled items certified to be free of pollutants and other contaminants.

Take alpha-lipoic acid, 100 to 400 milligrams a day. Note that this could possibly decreased blood glucose stages too much if the person getting drugs such as metformin - sufferers should work with their physicians so secure and proper dosages are employed.

The group of issues gathered under the heading metabolic problem does not seem to have one unique cause and does not involve a clear-cut target organ or system. For this reason, some researchers have considered whether it is necessary to separate out this particular group of conditions and give it the status of a problem. Most physicians, however, believe that the official identification of metabolic problem is validated.

Proponent's factor out that determining metabolic problem is a strong warning of wellness issues in a personal. In particular, if metabolic problem remains without treatment, the person is likely to create serious cardiac arrest and kind two diabetic issues.

The healthcare conditions in a personal with metabolic problem are complex and connected. However, the meaning of metabolic problem provides an obvious healing path for reducing an individual's possibility of creating center related illnesses and diabetic issues. All elements of metabolic problem can be treated by exercising, improving eating routine, and staying slim. In those cases where healing way of life changes are inadequate, the meaning of metabolic problem gives physicians a particular set of conditions (obesity, great blood pressure, dyslipidemias, and hyperinsulinemia) to treat independently.

Establishing metabolic problem as an enterprise also concentrates attention on certain key broken processes in the bodies of individuals who are on the road to serious wellness issues. Identifying the five conditions that write metabolic problem gives researchers essential objectives for studying, drug development, and healing advancement (Segal, pg. 76, 2008).
. At the same time, doctors caution that metabolic problem is a development of convenience. As currently described, metabolic problem is a excellent but not an ideal forecaster of the

possibility of creating serious wellness issues. Analysis continues, and it is likely that the meaning of metabolic problem will be customized later on.

A Formal Definition

Metabolic problem is not an illness in the usual sense. Instead, it is a situation, a collection of issues affecting the body ability to maintain flow of useful but not excessive energy elements (i.e., sugar and lipids) in the blood vessels. Initially, when these issues occur, they interact to intensify each other. Eventually, the set of issues becomes severe enough to lead to serious wellness repercussions. At this factor, physicians say that a personal has metabolic problem. It is still not obvious whether any one of the person issues of metabolic problem is the primary cause. More likely, two or more of the issues create independently and then set off the situation. In any case, current explanations are not based on cause. Instead, they have been designed by looking for groups of indicators in individuals who later designed center related illnesses or kind two diabetic issues.

From studies of large communities of individuals, the most typical group of signs has been discovered to consist of obesity, blood insulin resistance, dyslipidemia (either too much or too little fat in the blood), and great blood pressure. As of 2007, a globally accepted set of requirements for determining metabolic problem was still being worked out.

DEMOGRAPHICS

Is census helpful in acknowledging metabolic syndrome? The competition or gender of a personal that walks into the medical center is no help in determining whether that personal has metabolic problem. The individual's age is not much help, either. Senior citizens are more likely than youngsters to have the disorder, but 1 in 20 youngsters have metabolic problem. Occurrence does vary in different communities, but the problem is too typical everywhere to use census as a discriminator in medical practice.

Adolescents (12–19 years)

An approximated 2.9 million youngsters in the U. s. States—or 9.4% of those mature 12 to 19 years— have metabolic problem. It is more typical in teenage boys (13.2%) than in teenage girls (5.3%) and in Mexican-American (11.1%) and white-colored youngsters (10.7%) than in African-American youngsters (5.2%). Among obese or obese youngsters, the prevalence of metabolic problem is much higher: 44%.The requirements for analysis of metabolic problem in youngsters and children are modified for age.

Overweight youngsters who do not have metabolic problem remain at risk for creating it. Obesity—especially excess intra-abdominal fat—in childhood and puberty foreshadows unusually great blood vessels stages of blood insulin, triglycerides, and LDL cholesterol; low blood vessels stages of HDL cholesterol; and great blood pressure in maturity.

Adults (19 decades and older)

An approximated 35.1% of America men and 32.6% of America females have metabolic problem. The problem is more typical in seniors. It is discovered; for example, in 20.3% of men and 15.6% of females mature 20–39 decades. Among grownups mature 40–59 decades, the prevalence of metabolic problem improves to 40.8% in men and to 37.2% in females. The problem impacts more than half (51.5% of men, 54.4% of women) of People America mature 60 decades and mature (1).

Prevalence of metabolic problem differs considerably from nation to nation. This seems to be caused by two factors: (1) modifications in way of life (especially, diet, smoking, and level of actual exercise) between countries, and (2) modifications in competition. In all configurations and all communities, the prevalence of metabolic problem improves with age.

As in youngsters, the association of metabolic problem and race/ethnicity differs by sex. Among men, the approximated prevalence of metabolic problem is 37.2%, 25.3%, and 33.2% for white-colored People America, Africa People America, and Spanish People America, respectively. Among females, the corresponding rates are 31.5%, 38.8%, and 40.6% . Immigrant Oriental Indians in the U. s. States also have a great prevalence of metabolic problem, ranging from 26.9% (using the NCEP/ATP III definition) to 38.2% (IDF definition).

DIAGNOSING METABOLIC SYNDROME

Medical History

Diagnosing metabolic problem requires a actual evaluation and blood vessels assessments. However, the wellness background provides essential info that can confirm the analysis and help determine the extent of the problem.

A personal that has metabolic problem may already have been medically determined as having some elements of the problem, such as obesity, great blood pressure, or dyslipidemia. A significant problem of the problem (atherosclerotic artery illness, ischemic cardiac arrest, diabetes) may also be present.

In addition, the person may come with a analysis (or the signs and symptoms) of one of a number of other healthcare conditions that occur especially frequently with metabolic problem. Illnesses that are often discovered with metabolic problem include:

Gout: Almost sixty-six per cent of individuals with gouty arthritis have metabolic problem. Polycystic ovarian problem (PCOS): More than one third of females with PCOS have metabolic problem (Staels, pg. 97, 2009).

Wide spread lupus erythematosus (SLE): An approximated 16% to 32% of females with SLE have metabolic problem.

Fatty liver illness (Moore, 2010)

Serious renal disease

Osa or other rest interference disorders

Subclinical thyroid problems (low regular T4 levels)

Light intellectual incapacity in mature adults

Alzheimer's disease disease

Faster than regular prostate rate of growth in harmless prostatic hyperplasia (BPH)

Fibromyalgia

Cataracts

Two Key Physical Characteristics

When testing for metabolic problem, two actual dimensions must be included: hips area and great blood pressure.

INTRA-ABDOMINAL FAT

Today, the standard actual evaluation of a personal includes size and bodyweight but it does not usually consist of a statistic that is essential for detecting metabolic syndrome: the individual's hips area. Over the last 8 to 10 decades, it has been proven that the particular aspect of obesity that best alerts of upcoming heart issues is the amount of fat focused inside the stomach and hips area is an excellent evaluate of intra-abdominal fat (Grundy,pg97,2011).

Measuring Obesity

Obesity is a situation determined with having more saved human extra fat than is considered regular. Clinically, obesity is calculated ultimately. The simplest obesity tables compare two external actual measurements—height and weight—and obese is then described as "more than the regular bodyweight for a given size."

The most widely used evaluate of obesity is the bmi (BMI). This is calculated using the formula:

BMI = bodyweight in kgs / size in meters2

or

BMI = bodyweight in pounds x 703 / size in inches2

BMI has been proven to be a excellent oblique sign of the percentage of human extra fat, and it is the most widely used evaluate of total human extra fat.

If you suspect your individual has metabolic problem, acquire a individual record, including close relatives, personal, and public record to assess for diabetes; coronary, cerebral, and peripheral general disease; and genealogy of early cardiovascular illness and diabetic issues. Execute medication getting back together.

Ask the individual about his exercising. If he has a sedentary way of life, ask about actual limitations or aspects that might prohibit a rise in action stages. You'll also want to identify actual, emotional, or public limitations to way of life changes that he'll need to make to cure metabolic problem. Execute an actual assessment.

Obtain the individual's age, baseline hypertension, bodyweight, height, and determine his bmi (BMI). A BMI of 30 or higher indicates obesity; 25 to 29.9 is regarded overweight, and below 25 is the goal (however, a BMI below 18.5 is regarded underweight).

Take a hips statistic at the stage of the iliac crest at end-expiration. Be aware that minor increases in hips area (37 to 39 inches wide in men and 31 to 34 inches wide in women) put white, African-American, and Hispanic sufferers at increased threat for metabolic problem. Because the inherited contribution to blood insulin stage of resistance is strong in these sufferers, suggest way of life changes to decrease threat (McAllister, pg.98,2011).

Other tests for sufferers alleged of metabolic problem consist of a going on a fast lipid panel to assess triglycerides, and going on a fast lcd sugar stages. For sufferers with normal going on a fast sugar stages, an oral sugar tolerance test may be performed to detect prediabetes. A 2-hour lcd sugar of 140 to 199 mg/dL after a 75-gram sugar load enables as prediabetes (Mottillo, pg. 86,2010)

Treatment priorities

Although way of life changes can effectively cure metabolic problem, predisposing genetics also must be identified and addressed. Management of metabolic problem is aimed at slimming down and improving action, as these are the most effective interventions for decreasing blood insulin stage of resistance and decreasing abdominal area. The next therapeutic intervention is to initiate nutritional changes to decrease going on a fast sugar and triglyceride stages and enhance HDL cholesterol levels (Misra, pg25, 2011).

* To combat central being overweight, start the individual on a long-term losing bodyweight program. He should aim to lose 7% to 10% of complete bodyweight over the first year, with continued slow losing bodyweight thereafter until a BMI of 20 to 25 is reached. Rather than

decreasing calorie consumption drastically, he should decrease complete daily calorie consumption by 500 to 1,000 calorie consumption (Foster, pg. 50, 2011)

* Helping the individual's action stage can help decrease his chance of developing diabetic issues. The Finnish Diabetes Avoidance Research discovered that the overall occurrence of diabetic issues was reduced by 58% in sufferers whose way of life changes included losing bodyweight, decreasing nutritional fat consumption, improving soluble fiber, and participating in moderate exercise for at least 30 minutes a day (walking, biking, skiing, jogging, or swimming). Research topics also showed decreases in hypertension and triglyceride stages.3 These results were similar to those discovered in the Diabetes Avoidance Program Research, which looked at way of life changes vs. medication for decreasing the occurrence of type two diabetic issues.8 As with the Finnish study, topics who made way of life changes had a 58% decrease in the occurrence of diabetic issues. Subjects in the medication group had a 31% decrease in the development of diabetic issues (Makhsida, pg65, 2009),

* Blood vessels stress decrease may come about from making the recommended way of life changes, but if the individual's BP is still above 130/85 mm Hg, antihypertensive medication may be recommended to decrease the threat for general illness and center failure. The 7th Report of the Joint National Panel on Avoidance, Recognition, Evaluation, and Therapy of High Blood vessels Pressure (JNC 7), states that antihypertensive medications need to be recommended for sufferers with BPs of 140/90 or higher (130/80 or higher for those with diabetic issues or renal disease), and in sufferers for whom way of life changes haven't succeeded in reaching BP goals (Ulrig,pg87,2009)

* To correct dyslipidemia, way of life changes consist of replacing human extra fat with polyunsaturated human extra fat such as corn, soy bean, and sunflower sebum, and monounsaturated human extra fat such as canola, olive, and peanut sebum. Advise the individual to eat fish twice a week and follow the Dietary Approaches to Stop Hypertension

25

(DASH) diet to enhance triglyceride and blood choleseterol stages. Drug therapy may be needed, such as with statins, fibrates, and niacin (nicotinic acid) (Mendelson, pg100, 2008). Fibrate medication such as gemfibrozil and fenofibrate decrease triglyceride stages 20% to 50% and enhance HDL blood choleseterol stages by 10% to 20%. Statins consist of atorvastatin and lovastatin. Niacin preparations such as niasprin enhance HDL blood choleseterol stages by 15% to 35% and decrease triglyceride stages by 20% to 50%, but must be used very carefully and at lower amounts in sufferers with diabetic issues because of the potential to enhance sugar stages.7 Monitor the individual for muscle soreness, pain, and weakness, because fibrates and statins given in combination enhance the individual's threat for myopathies.

References

Friedman, M.. (2011). Specialized new graduate RN critical care orientation; retention and   financial impact. Journal of Nursing Economics, 29(1), 7-13.

Foster RR. (2011). The impact of a nursing transitions programme on retention and   cost savings. Journal of Nursing Management, 19, 50-6.

McAllister, M., Downer, T., Framp, A., Hanson, J., Cope, J., & Gamble, T. (2011). Building empathic practice through transformative learning theory. Australian Nursing Journal, 19(5), 22.

Mottillo S, Filion KB, Genest J, et al. (2010). The metabolic syndrome and cardiovascular risk.   A systematic review and meta-analysis. J Am Coll Cardiol, 56:1113-1132.

Bagchi, D. (2012). Nutritional and therapeutic interventions for diabetes and metabolic syndrome. Amsterdam: Elsevier/Academic Press.

Batone, T. E. (2008). Metabolic syndrome research trends. New York: Nova Science
Publishers.

Blaha, M. J. (2012). Metabolic syndrome from risk factors to management. Torino: SEEd.

Byrne, C. D. (2011). The metabolic syndrome (2nd ed.). Chichester, West Sussex: Wiley-
Blackwell.

Das, U. N. (2010). Metabolic syndrome pathophysiology: the role of essential fatty acids.
Ames, Iowa: Wiley-Blackwell.

Iacobellis, G. (2009). Drug-drug interactions in the metabolic syndrome. New York: Nova
Science Publishers.

Isaacs, S. (2010). Overcoming metabolic syndrome. Omaha, Neb.: Addicus Books.

Mendelson, S. D. (2008). Metabolic syndrome and psychiatric illness interactions,
pathophysiology, assessment and treatment. Amsterdam: Elsevier/Academic Press.

Misra, A. (2011). Recent advances in metabolic syndrome. Haryana: Elsevier.

Ulrig, G. T. (2009). Progress in metabolic syndrome research. New York: Nova Science
Publishers.

        Metabolic syndrome and mental illness." Harvard Mental Health Letter. 28(2):5
Aug. 2011

    "Can I reverse or slow the progression of metabolic syndrome through diet?" Duke
Medicine HealthNews, 17(5):8. May 2011

    "What is metabolic syndrome and how can it affect my heart health?" Duke Medicine
HealthNews, 16(10):8. Oct. 2010.

    "The physical activity, stress and metabolic syndrome triangle." Holmes ME. Obesity
Reviews, 11(7):492-507. July 2010.

        Endocrinology and Metabolism Clinics of North America. Metabolic Syndrome: Parts
I and II June 2004 and September 2004.

Hurst, RT, Lee, RW. Increased Incidence of Coronary Atheroscloerosis in Type 2 Diabetes Mellitus: Mechanisms and Management. Ann Intern Med 2010;139:824-834

Colhoun, JM, Betteridge, DJ, et al. Primary Prevention of Cardiovascular disease with Atorvastatin in Type 2 diabetes in the Collaborative Atorvastatin Diabetes Study (CARDS): Multicentre Randomized Placebo-controlled Trial. Lancet 2011;365-96

Weiss, R, Dziura, J, et al. Obesity and the Metabolic Syndrome in Children and Adolescents. NEJM 2012;350:2362-74

Abdul-Rahim, HF, Husseine, A, et al. The Metabolic Syndrome in the West Bank Population, An urban-rural comparison. Diabetes Care 2009;275-79

Vinik, AI, Natural History of the Metabolic Syndrome and Type 2 diabetes: The Ticking Clock. 65th Scientific Sessions of the American Diabetes Association. Diabetes Care 2012;275-79

Milionis, HJ, et al. Metabolic Syndrome Increases Stroke Risk in the Elderly. Stroke 2009;36:1372-1376

Segal, P, Zimmet, PZ, 1st International Congress on "Prediabetes" and the Metabolic Syndrome, April 13-16, 2005; Berlin, Germany. Medscape Diabetes &Endocrinology, 2008;7(2)

Staels, B, Fruchart, JC, Therapeutic Roles of Peroxisome Proliferator-Activated Receptor Agonists. Diabetes 2009;54(8):2460-2470

Makhsida, N, Shah, J, et al. Hypogonadism and Metabolic Syndromne: Implications for Testosterone Therapy. J Urol. 2009 Sept;174(3):827-34

(1)Peters, Anne, The Broadening Domain of the Metabolic Syndrdome. 65th Scientific Session of the American Diabetes Association.

Kahn, R, Buse, J, et al. The Metabolic Syndrome: Time for a Critical Appraisal. Diabetes Care 2005;28:2289-2304

(3)Shulman, A, Mangelsdorf, D, Retinoid X Receptor Heterodimers in the Metabolic Syndrome. NEJM 2005; 353:604 -15

(2)Program and Abstracts of the 65th Scientific Sessions of the American Diabetes Association; June 10-14, 2005; San Diego, California

Redmon, JB, Raatz, SK, et al. Two-year outcome of a combination of weight loss therapies for subjects with type 2 diabetes: a randomized trial. Diabetes Care. 2012;28:1311-1315

Domanski,M, Mitchell, G, et al. Pulse pressure and cardiovascular disease-related mortality: follow-up study of the Multiple Risk Factor Intervention Trial (MRFIT). JAMA. 2002 May 22-29;287(20):2666-2830

Sytkowski, PA, D'agostino, RB, et al. Secular trends in long-term sustained hypertension, long-term treatment and cardiovascular mortality. The Framingham Heart Study 1950-1990. Circulation 1996 Feb.15;93(4):697-703

Redmon, JB, Reck, KP, et al. Two-year outcome of a combination of weight loss therapies for type 2 diabetes. Diabetes Care 2005;28:1311-1315

Eurich, DT, Majumdar, SR, et al. Improved clinical outcomes associated with metformin in patients with diabetes and heart failure. Diabetes Care 2005;28:2345-2351

Gillespie, EL, White, CM, et al. The impact of ACE inhibitors or Angiotensin II receptor blockers on the development of new-onset type 2 diabetes. Diabetes Care 2005; 28:2261-2266

American Diabetes Association: Clinical Practice Recommendations 2005. Diabetes Care, January 2005;28:Supplement

Cornier MA, Dabelea D, Hernandez TL, et al. The metabolic syndrome. Endocr Rev. 2008;29:777-822.Ford ES, Giles WH, Dietz WH.

(4) Prevalence of the metabolic syndrome among US adults: findings from the third National Health and Nutrition Examination Survey. JAMA. 2002;287:356-359.

Reaven G. Metabolic syndrome: pathophysiology and implications for management of cardiovascular disease. Circulation. 2002;106:286-288.

Park YW, Zhu S, Palaniappan L, et al. The metabolic syndrome: prevalence and associated risk factor findings in the US population from the Third National Health and Nutrition Examination Survey, 1988-1994. Arch Intern Med. 2003;163:427-436

Wang H, Dong S, Xu H, et al. Genetic variants in FTO associa ted with metabolic syndrome: a meta- and gene-based analysis. Mol Biol Rep. 2012;39:5691-5698.

Grundy SM, Brewer HB Jr, Cleeman JI, et al; American Heart Association; National Heart, Lung, and Blood Institute. Definition of metabolic syndrome: report of the National Heart, Lung, and Blood Institute/American Heart Association conference on scientific issues related to definition. Circulation. 2009;109:433-438.

Athyros VG, Ganotakis E, Kolovou GD, et al. Assessing the treatment effect in metabolic syndrome without perceptible diabetes (ATTEMPT): a prospective-randomized study in middle aged men and women. Curr Vasc Pharmacol. 2011;9:647-657.

(6) National Cholesterol Education Program (NCEP) Expert Panel on Detection, Evaluation, and Treatment of High Blood Cholesterol in Adults (Adult Treatment Panel III). Third report of the National Cholesterol Education Program (NCEP) Expert Panel on Detection, Evaluation, and Treatment of High Blood Cholesterol in Adults (Adult Treatment Panel III) final report. Circulation. 2002;106:3143-3421.